SOURSOP; NATURE'S GIFT.

Unlocking The Anticancer Properties, Numerous Health and Nutritional Benefits of Soursop.

Odane Alvaro

Table Of Contents.

Introduction

Chapter 1

Origin and Historical Significance of Soursop.

    1.1 Overview of Soursop

    1.2 Nutritional Composition of Soursop.

    1.3 Phytochemicals and Antioxidants in Soursop.

Chapter 2

Medicinal uses/Health Benefits of Soursop.

    2.1 Anticancer Properties of Soursop.

    2.2 Digestive Health

    2.3 Soursop and Heart Health

    2.4 Soursop and its Impact on Mental Well-being

Chapter 3

Soursop in Skincare and Haircare.

    3.1 Slowing Down Aging Processes

Chapter 4

Soursop Products and Supplements.

    4.1 Tea and Infusions.

    4.2 Fresh Soursop Recipes

    4.3 Supplements and Extracts

Conclusion

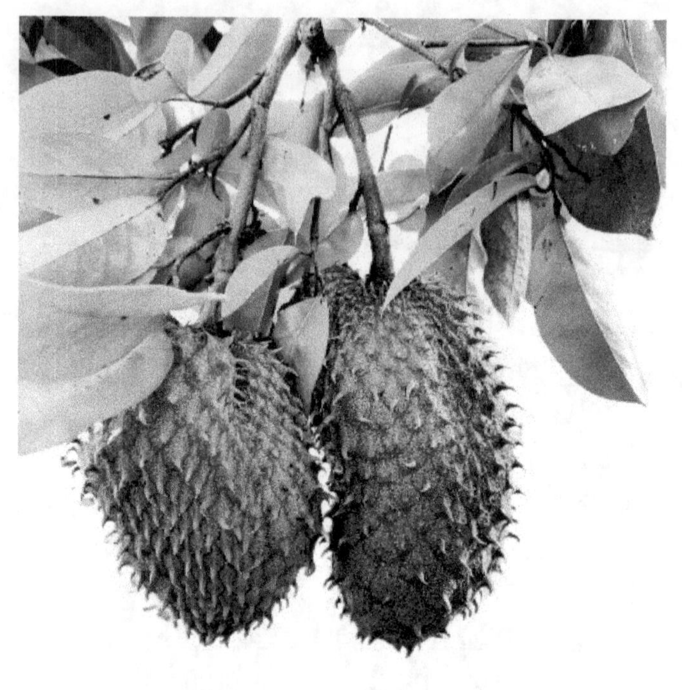

Introduction.

In the lush tropical areas of the world, tucked away in luxuriant vegetation is the wonderful fruit known as soursop. The soursop hides a magical secret inside that is just waiting to be unlocked. From its flavorful, custard-like flesh, to the depths of its vibrant green exterior.

Scientifically known as Annona muricata, soursop has fascinated cultures all over the world for centuries with its unique flavor, captivating look, and outstanding health benefits. Although originally from the tropical Americas, soursop has crossed geographical boundaries to become a popular and sought-after fruit all across the world.

Soursop has earned a special position in traditional medicine, with its many parts and extracts being used for their possible medicinal powers. Soursop has been praised for its potential as a natural cure for a variety of diseases, from boosting the immune system to aiding healthy digestion. We investigate the science underlying its extraordinary qualities and how it has been utilized as a powerful cure for a variety of illnesses.

Join me as I solve the mysteries and reveal the abundance of this remarkable fruit. You are about to go on a journey that will leave you absolutely charmed with the delights of this magnificent fruit, from its exotic origins to its tantalizing taste. Let us unlock the sour power together and explore the hidden treasures of the soursop.

Chapter 1

Origin and Historical Significance of Soursop.

1.1 Overview of Soursop.

The soursop fruit, scientifically known as Annona muricata, has a long history spanning centuries and cultures. It is known as Guanábana in Hispanic America. In Indonesia, it is known as Sirsak. Soursop, which is native to the Americas and the Caribbeans, has played a diverse role in numerous communities throughout history, leaving an unmistakable impact on culinary traditions, medicinal, and cultural customs.

Indigenous tribes in South and Central America have long cherished soursop as a precious fruit with legendary and spiritual significance. It was frequently thought to be a symbol of fertility, abundance, and vigor. The fruit's distinct look, with its spiky green covering and creamy flesh, captivated early civilizations, who believed it possessed supernatural properties.

The historical significance of soursop in traditional medicine is particularly notable. Native tribes regarded the fruit as therapeutic and used it to treat a variety of diseases. Its leaves, bark, roots, and fruit were used to treat fevers, digestive problems, parasite infections, and even as a sedative. These ancient medicinal methods were eventually passed down through generations, and they had an impact on the development of herbal medicine in many places.

Soursop traveled beyond its home countries and reached new coasts throughout the era of exploration. During their conquests of the Americas, Spanish conquistadors found the fruit and brought it back to Europe. Its arrival prompted curiosity and attention, resulting in its establishment in a number of European colonies and gardens. The exotic charm and refreshing flavor of soursop quickly became popular among European aristocrats.

Soursop gained a place in the culinary traditions of various cultures as it traveled across continents. Soursop, for example, became a popular ingredient in cooling beverages, ice creams, and desserts throughout the Caribbean. It was used in traditional Asian meals and herbal teas, bringing a pleasant tanginess and scent to the cuisine. Soursop is referred to as "Hanuman Phal" in India and "Mullaatha" in Sri Lanka. Soursop has been utilized in Ayurvedic medicine, India's traditional medical system, for its cooling effects and as a cure for digestive issues, fever, inflammation, and skin conditions.

Soursop continues to amaze and inspire people today. Its historical significance as a fruit inextricably linked to human culture, health, and culinary activities attests to its enduring attractiveness. As we explore further into its mysteries and uncover its potential, Soursop remains an intriguing fruit that bridges the gap between our ancient history and our modern appreciation for nature's gifts.

While the soursop tree is a single species, Annona muricata, there are multiple recognized variants or cultivars of soursop that have minimal differences in taste, size, and texture. Here are some prominent types of soursop:

- **Morada(Brazil):** The Morada type is well-known for its huge size and vivid purple skin. Its flesh is creamy, white, and succulent, with a characteristic tangy-sweet flavor. Morada soursops are prized for their great flavor and eye-catching appearance.

- **Fibreless Cuban (Australia):** As the name implies, this soursop variety is characterized by a lack of fibers in the flesh, resulting in a smooth and velvety feel. The lack of fiber makes it especially tempting to people who want a more luxurious diet.

- **Bennett**: The Bennett soursop cultivar is native to Jamaica and is prized for its rich flavor. It has a delicate balance of sweetness and acidity, as well as a smooth and velvety texture. Bennett soursop is often utilized in the preparation of soursop-based beverages and sweets.

1.2 Nutritional Composition of Soursop.

Soursop has around 16.8 grams of carbs per 100 grams. These carbohydrates are mostly sugars like glucose and fructose. Soursop has a relatively high natural sugar content, which adds to its sweet flavor. Soursop is high in fiber. This fiber level can help with regular bowel motions and overall digestive health. The following is an approximate nutritional

breakdown per 100 grams of soursop
fruit:

Calories: 66

Carbohydrates: 16.8 grams

Dietary Fiber: 3.3 grams

Protein: 1 gram

Fat: 0.3 grams

Vitamin C: 20.6 milligrams (34% of the
daily recommended intake)

Potassium: 278 milligrams

Magnesium: 21 milligrams

Calcium: 14 milligrams

Iron: 0.6 milligrams

Vitamin B1 (Thiamine): 0.07 milligrams

Vitamin B2 (Riboflavin): 0.05 milligrams

Vitamin B3 (Niacin): 0.9 milligrams

Vitamin B6: 0.06 milligrams.

It's worth noting that the nutritional
makeup of soursop varies slightly
depending on ripeness and other factors.
Soursop also contains antioxidants,

which are helpful molecules that protect the body from free radicals and oxidative stress. These antioxidants, which include acetogenins, flavonoids, and phenolic substances, may contribute to the potential health benefits of eating soursop.

1.3 Phytochemicals and Antioxidants in Soursop.

Soursop has a variety of phytochemicals, which are natural components found in plants that contribute to its color, flavor, and potential health benefits. Soursop phytochemicals have received interest due to their possible antioxidant, anti-inflammatory, and anticancer effects. Soursop contains the following significant phytochemicals:

Acetogenins: Soursop is high in acetogenins, a type of phytochemical found only in the Annonaceae family of plants. These chemicals have been researched for their anticancer effects and are thought to impede the growth of specific cancer cells.

Flavonoids: Flavonoids found in soursop include quercetin, kaempferol, and rutin. Flavonoids have antioxidant and anti-inflammatory effects, which may help protect cells from free radical damage and reduce inflammation in the body.

Phenolic compounds: Soursop includes phenolic components such as tannins and phenolic acids, which have antioxidant and anti-inflammatory properties. These chemicals aid in the scavenging of free radicals and the protection of cells from oxidative stress.

Vitamin C: While not strictly a phytochemical, vitamin C is a potent antioxidant present in soursop. It is essential for immune system support, collagen formation, and cell protection from oxidative damage.

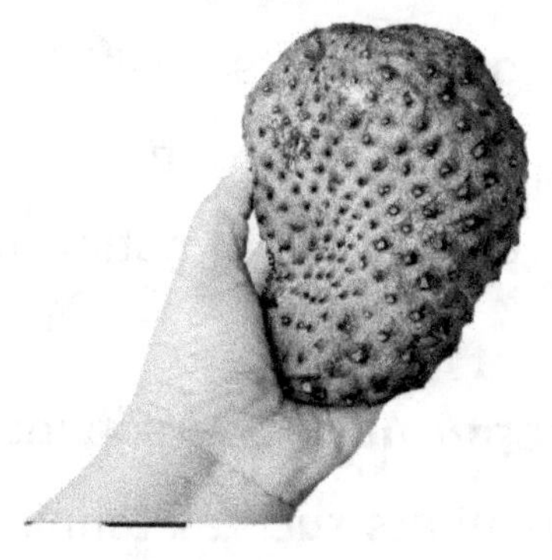

Chapter 2

Medicinal Uses/Health Benefits of Soursop.

Soursop has been used for generations for its therapeutic benefits, in addition to its delectable taste. It is thought to have multiple health benefits and has been examined for its possible use in a variety of medical disorders. Soursop is high in vitamin C, which is believed to help the immune system. Soursop consumption may assist to boost the immune system and defend against common illnesses and infections. Because of its anti-inflammatory characteristics, soursop has traditionally been used to treat inflammation-related diseases such as arthritis and joint pain.

2.1 Anticancer Properties of Soursop.

Soursop's anticancer activities are mostly ascribed to its high phytochemical composition, which contains acetogenins, alkaloids, flavonoids, polyphenols, and annonaceous acetogenins. Several researchers have looked at these chemicals and their impact on cancer cells, with promising results. Here are some of the primary ways that soursop has been related to anticancer effects:

- **Antioxidant Properties:** Soursop contains significant levels of antioxidants, which play an important role in neutralizing free radicals, which can harm cells and lead to cancer growth. Antioxidants protect cells from oxidative stress, which has been linked to cancer start and progression.

- **Cytotoxic Effects:** Extracts from several sections of the soursop plant, particularly the leaves and fruit, have been demonstrated in studies to have cytotoxic effects against cancer cells. Cytotoxicity refers to the ability to cause cell death in cancer cells while sparing healthy cells, which is required for prospective cancer therapies.

- **Apoptosis Induction:** Soursop extracts have been shown to induce apoptosis, also known as programmed cell death, in cancer cells. Apoptosis is a natural process that aids in the elimination of damaged or abnormal cells, and its disturbance can lead to the development of cancer. The capacity of soursop to cause apoptosis in cancer cells is viewed as a promising method in cancer treatment.

- **Anti-Angiogenic Effects:** Soursop extracts have anti-angiogenic effects, which means they can block the creation of new blood vessels that deliver nutrition and oxygen to tumors. Soursop can slow tumor development and spread by blocking the tumor's blood supply.

- **Inhibition of Cancer Cell Proliferation:** Studies have shown that soursop extracts can limit the growth and division of cancer cells. This impact is critical in preventing metastasis and managing cancer progression.

- **Immune System Stimulation:** Some study suggests that soursop may boost immune system activity, allowing it to better recognize and target cancer cells. A strong immune response is critical in fighting cancer and preventing recurrence.

In summary, soursop has various potentially helpful anticancer characteristics due to its diverse array of bioactive chemicals.

2.2 Digestive Health.

Soursop's high fiber content is one of its important components that aids in digestive health. Fiber is essential for maintaining regular bowel movements and avoiding constipation. It provides mass to the stool, allowing it to travel more efficiently through the intestines. Soursop can help prevent digestive disorders including bloating, gas, and discomfort by encouraging regularity.

Furthermore, the fiber in soursop functions as a probiotic, providing food for the good bacteria in the gut. Probiotic bacteria serve an important part in maintaining a healthy gut microbiota. A healthy gut microbiome improves digestion, nutrient absorption, and immunological function. Soursop has natural enzymes and chemicals that aid in digestion. For example, it contains high levels of fiber-digesting enzymes such as cellulase and hemicellulase. These enzymes degrade complex carbs and aid in their absorption.

- **Alleviating Gastric Pain:** Soursop's analgesic properties may help ease the discomfort and agony associated with gastritis. Soursop's natural chemicals may provide relief by acting on pain receptors and lowering pain perception.

- **Soursop and Acid Reflux:** Acid reflux occurs when stomach acid runs back into the esophagus, producing heartburn, regurgitation, and discomfort. The alkaline composition of soursop may assist to control stomach acid levels. Soursop may help ease symptoms of acid reflux and create a more comfortable digestive experience by lowering excessive acidity. Soursop's anti-inflammatory qualities may help calm the irritated esophageal lining produced by acid reflux. Soursop may help to treat acid reflux symptoms by lowering inflammation.

- **Antimicrobial Properties:** Soursop contains natural antibacterial qualities that can aid in the fight against dangerous bacteria and parasites in the digestive system. Certain chemicals contained in soursop, such as acetogenins and alkaloids, have been demonstrated in studies to have antibacterial activity against a variety of pathogens, including bacteria and parasites that can cause gastrointestinal infections.

Soursop may help restore the natural balance of the gut microbiota and create a healthy digestive environment by inhibiting the growth of dangerous microbes. Incorporating soursop into your diet can bring considerable digestive health advantages. It is a helpful addition due to its high fiber content, digestive enzymes, antibacterial qualities, and anti-inflammatory effects.

2.3 Soursop and Heart Health

Heart disease is still the top cause of death worldwide, emphasizing the significance of keeping a healthy cardiovascular system. While regular exercise and a balanced diet are important lifestyle variables, nature has also endowed us with specific fruits and plants that may offer considerable benefits for heart health. We will investigate the potential of soursop in boosting cardiovascular health.

Soursop is a nutritious powerhouse as well as a tasty tropical fruit. It is rich in vitamins and minerals like vitamin C, vitamin B6, fiber, potassium, and magnesium. These nutrients, as well as the presence of bioactive substances, contribute to soursop's possible cardiovascular advantages.

- **Blood Pressure Regulation:** High blood pressure, often known as hypertension, is a major risk factor for cardiovascular disease. Soursop's potassium concentration is significant in this regard. Potassium is a necessary mineral that aids in blood pressure regulation by counteracting the effects of sodium, a mineral that can lead to excessive blood pressure. As part of a balanced diet, eating potassium-rich foods like soursop may help maintain healthy blood pressure levels and lessen the load on the cardiovascular system. Individuals with kidney difficulties or those on medications that influence potassium levels, on the other hand, should consult with their healthcare provider before increasing their potassium intake.

- **Cholesterol Management:** Elevated LDL (low-density lipoprotein) cholesterol levels, sometimes known as "bad" cholesterol, lead to atherosclerosis and raise the risk of heart disease. Dietary options that properly regulate cholesterol levels are critical to heart health. The fibre content of soursop, particularly soluble fibre, may help with cholesterol management. Soluble fibre aids in the reduction of cholesterol absorption from the digestive tract, resulting in decreased LDL cholesterol levels.

Individuals can help manage their cholesterol levels and minimize their risk of heart disease by integrating soursop into a heart-healthy diet.

Soursop offers promise as a healthy fruit for heart health due to its antioxidant capacity, blood pressure regulation potential, cholesterol management qualities, and anti-inflammatory benefits. It's crucial to note, however, that a well-rounded approach to cardiovascular health should include other lifestyle factors like frequent exercise, maintaining a healthy weight, and avoiding tobacco use.

2.4 Soursop and its Impact on Mental Well-being.

In addition to its physical health advantages, Soursop has received attention for its possible favorable impact on mental well-being. Soursop's distinct combination of nutrients and bioactive substances contributes to its potential as a natural help in the promotion of mental health and overall psychological well-being. We'll look at the connection between soursop and mental health, concentrating on how it affects mood, stress, and cognitive performance.

- **Soursop and Mood Enhancement:** Mood disorders such as sadness and anxiety can have a substantial impact on a person's quality of life. Soursop has a number of chemicals that have been shown to improve mood and reduce symptoms associated with certain diseases.

- **Serotonin Boost:** Soursop contains tryptophan, an amino acid that is required for the creation of serotonin, a neurotransmitter known as the "feel-good" hormone. Serotonin is essential for mood regulation, and low levels of serotonin are linked to depression and anxiety. Soursop may support the creation of serotonin by providing the essential precursor, potentially enhancing mood and overall well-being.

- **Anti-Anxiety Effects:** In animal experiments, some chemicals contained in soursop, such as annonacin and flavonoids, have demonstrated potential anxiolytic qualities. These substances may aid in the reduction of anxiety symptoms by altering neurotransmitter activity in the brain and producing a sensation of peace and relaxation.

- **Soursop and Stress Reduction:** Chronic stress can be harmful to both mental and physical health. The natural components of soursop may assist to reduce the effects of stress on the body.

- **Adaptogenic Potential:** Soursop can help the body better adapt to and cope with stress. Adaptogens reduce the harmful physiological and psychological effects of prolonged stress by modulating the release of stress hormones such as cortisol.

- **Calming Effects:** Soursop's bioactive components, including acetogenins and flavonoids, have been shown to have sedative and relaxing properties. These characteristics may benefit in stress management by relaxing the mind, reducing restlessness, and promoting a sense of tranquility.

- **Soursop and Cognitive Function:** The unique components of soursop may have potential cognitive function and memory enhancing benefits.

- **Neuroprotective Properties:** Soursop contains antioxidants that protect brain cells from oxidative stress and free radical damage. This protection may help to preserve cognitive function and lower the likelihood of neurodegenerative disorders like Alzheimer's and Parkinson's.

- **Improved Brain Circulation:** Soursop has chemicals that may improve blood circulation in the brain. Improved blood flow to the brain promotes adequate oxygen and nutrition availability, promoting optimal brain function and cognition. Soursop is a fascinating natural aid in enhancing mental health due to its capacity to improve mood, reduce stress, and support cognitive function.

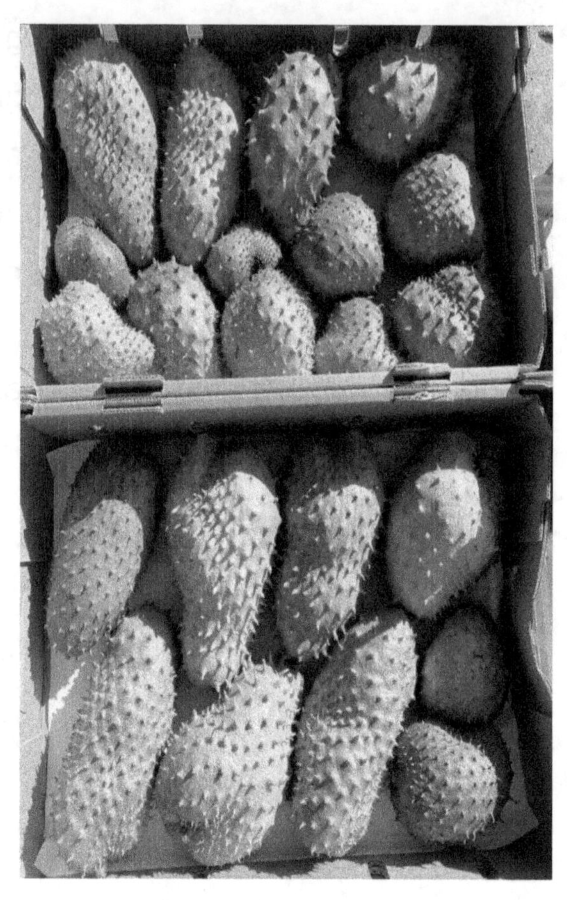

Chapter 3

Soursop in Skincare and Haircare.

As we attempt to keep our young appearance and vitality, the search for natural anti-aging therapies continues. The extraordinary soursop is one such potential answer. Soursop has been lauded for its several health advantages, including anti-aging potential.

3.1 Slowing Down Aging Processes

Before getting into the unique anti-aging benefits of soursop, it is critical to first understand the basic causes of aging. Aging is a multifaceted process that is influenced by both genetic and environmental variables. Oxidative stress, which arises when there is an imbalance between the generation of harmful free radicals and the body's ability to neutralize them with antioxidants, is a major contributor to aging. This imbalance, over time, causes cellular damage, inflammation, and the beginning of age-related disorders.

Soursop, being an antioxidant-rich food, plays an important function in countering oxidative stress. Antioxidants destroy free radicals and safeguard our cells from damage, slowing down the aging process. Soursop contains a variety of antioxidants, including vitamin C, vitamin E, beta-carotene, and phytochemicals such as acetogenins, annonaceous acetogenins, and flavonoids.

- **Vitamin C:** Soursop is high in vitamin C, a powerful antioxidant that protects the skin from free radical damage induced by exposure to environmental factors such as pollution and UV radiation. Vitamin C also stimulates collagen synthesis, a protein that keeps the skin's suppleness and firmness, decreasing the appearance of wrinkles and fine lines.

- **Vitamin E:** Soursop is also composed of vitamin E, a fat-soluble antioxidant that prevents oxidative damage to cell membranes. Vitamin E helps to maintain the integrity of the skin by neutralizing free radicals, thus preventing premature aging.

Our skin's health frequently reflects the aging process. The antioxidant qualities of soursop can benefit skin health by promoting a young appearance and preventing common indicators of aging. Here are a few ways that soursop might help your skin:

- **Wrinkle Reduction:** The high vitamin C concentration of soursop increases collagen formation, which reduces the appearance of wrinkles and fine lines, giving the skin a smoother and more youthful appearance.
- **Skin Hydration:** Soursop has natural components that help the skin retain moisture, avoiding dryness and improving overall hydration. Proper hydration is critical for skin elasticity and suppleness.
- **Skin Regeneration:** The antioxidants in soursop can help with skin cell regeneration, repairing damaged tissues, and contributing to a more youthful and vibrant complexion.

Soursop's high antioxidant content, which includes vitamin C, vitamin E, acetogenins, and flavonoids, makes it a promising natural therapy for anti-aging. Soursop may help retain a youthful appearance and promote general well-being by countering oxidative stress, decreasing inflammation, and maintaining healthy skin. Consuming soursop or utilising skincare products containing soursop extract may provide you with the anti-aging advantages that this wonderful fruit provides. However, it is important to remember that soursop should be used in moderation, and checking with a healthcare practitioner before making any changes is advised.

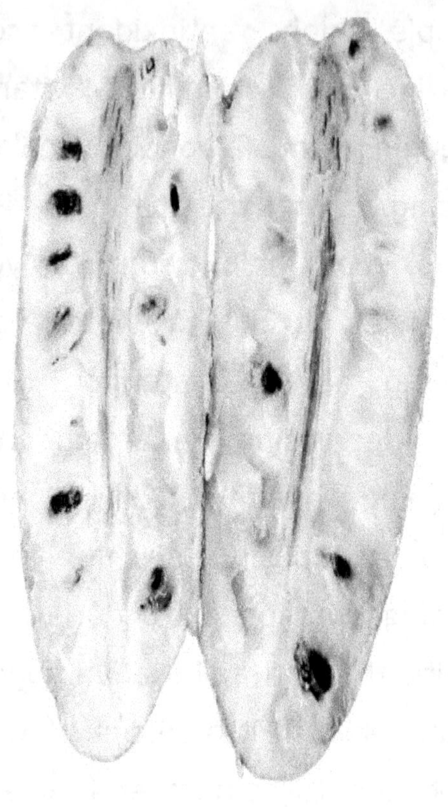

Chapter 4

Soursop Products and Supplements.

4.1 Tea and Infusions.

Follow these instructions to make tea using soursop leaves.

- **Gather the following ingredients:**

Fresh or dried soursop leaves

Sweetener (honey, sugar, or stevia) optional.

Water

- **Clean the soursop leaves:**

When using fresh soursop leaves, thoroughly wash them under running water to remove any dirt or contaminants.

If you're using dried soursop leaves, make sure they're clean and clear of debris.

- **Boil the water:**

Measure the amount of water needed based on how many cups of tea you wish to make and boil.

- **Add the soursop leaves:**

When the water is boiling, add the soursop leaves to the pot.
Use 2-3 soursop leaves per cup of water.

- **Simmer the leaves:**

Reduce the heat to low and allow the soursop leaves simmer in the water for about 10 minutes. Simmering the leaves allows the tastes and beneficial components to seep into the water.

- **Strain the tea:**

Remove the pot from the heat after it has begun to simmer.

Separate the tea from the soursop leaves using a fine-mesh sieve or a tea strainer. Throw away the leaves or compost them.

To improve the flavor, you can add a sweetener such as honey, sugar, or stevia.

Stir thoroughly to ensure that the sweetener is completely dissolved.

4.2 Fresh Soursop Recipes.

Consume the ripe fruit to enjoy soursop in its natural state. Simply cut up the soursop, remove the seeds, and enjoy the creamy, sweet flesh. To properly regulate calorie intake, remember to control portion sizes. Here are some delicious recipes that make use of soursop:

- **Soursop Smoothies:** Blend fresh soursop with low-fat yogurts or a plant-based milk substitute like almond milk or coconut milk. For an added nutritional boost, add a handful of spinach or kale. Smoothies can be a filling and satisfying low-calorie supper or snack.

Ingredients:

1 cup fresh soursop pulp (without seeds)

1 banana, ripe

1 cup canned coconut milk

1 teaspoon honey or maple syrup

Half teaspoon of vanilla extract

Ice cubes are optional.

Instructions:

1. Blend the soursop pulp, ripe banana, coconut milk, honey (or maple syrup), and vanilla essence in a blender.

2. Blend until the mixture is smooth

3. Add a few ice cubes if desired for a chilly smoothie.

4. Pour the tropical delight into glasses and enjoy.

- **Soursop Sorbet:**

Ingredients:

2 cups fresh soursop pulp (seeds removed)

1/2 cup sugar

1/4 cup water

1 tablespoon lime or lemon juice

Instructions:

1. In a small saucepan, mix the sugar and water. Stir constantly over medium heat until the sugar melts completely. Allow the syrup to cool.

2. Blend the soursop pulp and lime or lemon juice in a blender until smooth.

3. Mix together the soursop puree and the cooled sugar syrup.

4. Fill an ice cream maker halfway with the mixture and churn according to the manufacturer's directions until it reaches sorbet consistency.

5. Freeze the sorbet in an airtight container for a few hours before serving.

- **Skewers of Grilled Soursop Shrimp:**

Ingredients:

1 pound large shrimp, peeled and deveined

1 cup fresh soursop pulp (seeds removed)

2 tablespoons olive oil

2 cloves garlic, minced

1 teaspoon grated ginger

1 tablespoon lime juice

1 teaspoon honey

Salt and pepper to taste

Skewers (soak in water if using wooden skewers)

Instructions:

1. Combine the soursop pulp, olive oil, minced garlic, grated ginger, lime juice, honey, salt, and pepper in a mixing bowl to make the marinade.

2. Pour the marinade over the peeled and deveined shrimp, making sure they are equally coated. Refrigerate the bowl for at least 30 minutes after it has been covered.

3. Preheat the grill to medium-high temperature.

4. Thread the skewers with the marinated shrimp.

5. Grill the shrimp skewers for about 2-3 minutes per side, or until

cooked through and slightly browned.

Grilled soursop shrimp skewers go well with rice or a fresh salad.

- **Soursop Salad:** To make a refreshing salad, combine chopped soursop with other low-calorie fruits such as berries or citrus segments. For added taste, sprinkle with mint leaves or squeeze with some lime juice.

These soursop recipes are only a taste of the delicious options that this versatile fruit provides. Whether you prefer it in sweet or savory dishes, Soursop's distinct flavour will keep you wanting more. Experiment with various methods to incorporate soursop into your meals and snacks to enjoy its distinct flavour while keeping a healthy calorie balance. Bon appétit.

4.3 Supplements and Extracts.

- **Soursop Capsules:** Soursop capsules are an easy way to get soursop extract. They often contain a concentrated version of soursop extract, delivering a standardized amount of soursop's active components. Individuals who find it difficult to swallow fresh soursop or prefer a more concentrated form of the fruit's therapeutic components frequently prefer capsules.

- **Soursop Powder:** Soursop Powder is created by drying and grinding the fruit or its extracts into a fine powder. It can be used in smoothies, drinks, and other culinary preparations, making it simple to incorporate into one's diet. Many of the nutritional components and potential health advantages of fresh soursop are retained in soursop powder.

- **Soursop Liquid Extracts:** Soursop liquid extracts are concentrated versions of the active chemicals found in the fruit. They're usually prepared by extracting the beneficial components of soursop with a solvent like water or alcohol. Liquid extracts are versatile since they can be mixed into beverages, used as flavorings, or consumed straight.

It is important to choose soursop supplements or extracts from trustworthy suppliers who adhere to quality standards and efficiently source their ingredients. Follow the manufacturer's recommended dose directions or contact with a healthcare professional for specific guidance. Dosage may vary depending on factors such as age, health condition, and desired advantages. While soursop is typically safe to consume, some people may develop allergic reactions or stomach discomfort. Before using soursop supplements or extracts, speak with a healthcare practitioner if you have any known sensitivities or medical issues. Soursop supplements and extracts provide a handy and concentrated way to acquire soursop's possible health advantages. Soursop supplements, whether in the form of capsules, powders, or liquid extracts, can give antioxidants, immunological support, anti-inflammatory qualities, and digestive health benefits. Finally, to guarantee safe and appropriate use, it is critical to select high-quality goods, adhere to recommended dosages, and speak with a healthcare practitioner. Remember that supplements should enhance, not replace, a healthy diet and lifestyle.

Conclusion.

In this extensive survey of the benefits of soursop (Annona muricata), we delved into the extraordinary qualities of this tropical fruit and its possible impact on our health and well-being. Soursop has emerged as an essential asset to our search for maximum health, from its rich nutritional profile to its antioxidant power and different medicinal characteristics. Throughout this book, we've discovered that soursop contains a wealth of vital vitamins, minerals, and dietary fiber that contribute to overall nutrition. Its antioxidant capabilities, which include the presence of vitamin C, vitamin E, flavonoids, and other bioactive substances, help protect our cells from oxidative stress and maintain a healthy immune system.

Furthermore, the scientific world is excited about soursop's potential as an anticancer drug. Preliminary findings indicate that soursop may contain chemicals that impede cancer cell proliferation, presenting a promising option for future therapeutic improvements.

In addition, we explored how soursop can benefit digestive health, potentially providing treatment for stomach problems such as ulcers, gastritis, and acid reflux. Its anti-inflammatory and protective characteristics have shown effectiveness in lowering inflammation, protecting the stomach lining, and creating a healthier gastrointestinal tract. Soursop has been shown to improve emotional well-being in addition to physical health. Compounds like tryptophan and antioxidants may be responsible for its capacity to enhance mood, alleviate stress, and promote cognitive function. As we wrap off our look at the benefits of soursop, it's important to realize that, while it shows promise, it's not a magic cure-all. It should be regarded as a helpful addition to a well-balanced diet and a healthy lifestyle, supplementing other well-established practices for overall well-being. To ensure safe and optimal usage, it is important to check with healthcare specialists, when contemplating soursop supplements or extracts, especially for persons with underlying health concerns or those using drugs.

Finally, soursop is a tribute to the miracles that nature delivers. Its nutritional content, antioxidant power, anticancer potential, digestive health support, and beneficial impact on mental well-being make it a fruit worth exploring and incorporating into our life. May the information in this book help you make informed health decisions, and may the benefits of soursop help you on your way to a healthier, happier life. Appreciate the promise of soursop and go on a path of well-being inspired by nature's offerings.

www.ingramcontent.com/pod-product-compliance
Lightning Source LLC
Chambersburg PA
CBHW060214260726
48658CB00005BA/2034